Renal Diet Cookbook - Snacks and Desserts

52 Easy, Mouthwatering Snacks and Desserts Recipes that Include Sodium, Potassium and Phosphorous Amounts

Sabrina Sharp

Contents

Introduction

It is important to eat a wide variety of foods to stay healthy and strong. If you have kidney issues, then you are also advised to change your diet so as to consume smaller quantities of potassium, sodium, and phosphorous. This diet is referred to as the *renal diet*. Since everyone is different, patients with malfunctioning kidneys will have different dietary requirements to abide by. To get a meal plan that works for you, speak to a renal dietitian (a diet and nutrition consultant for people with kidney disease). A kidney-friendly diet will also help you protect your kidneys from further damage.

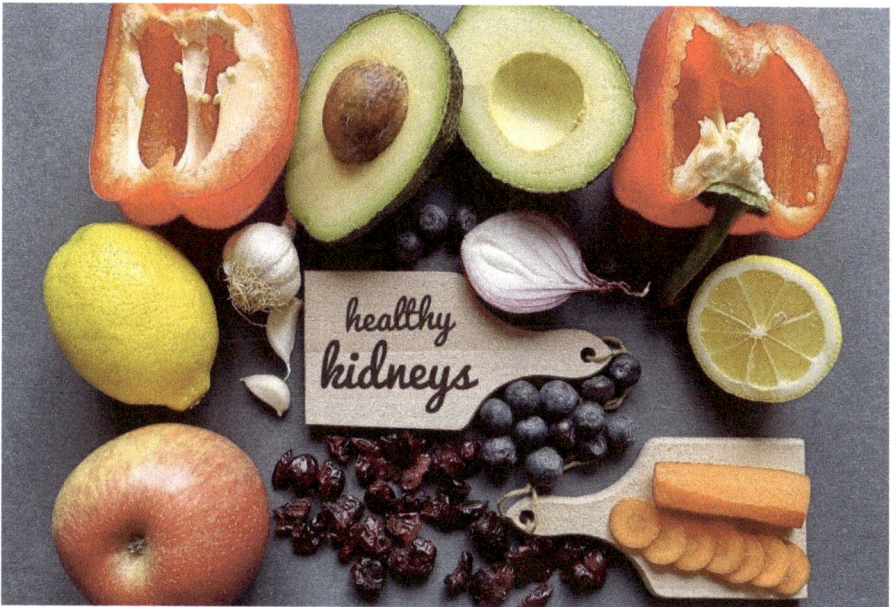

Snacks & Beverages

1. Hot Turkey Wings

Preparation time: 50 mins

Servings: 7

Ingredients

- 7 whole turkey wings
- 2 tsps. hot chili powder
- 2 tsps. garlic powder
- 2 tsps. onion powder
- 1 1/2 cups reduced-sodium barbecue sauce
- 1 tsp. smoked paprika
- 1 tsp. red pepper flakes
- 1 tsp. black pepper
- 1 cup brown sugar

Nutritional facts per serving

- Calories: 273cal
- Fat: 3g
- Sodium: 372mg
- Protein: 20g
- Potassium: 322mg
- Phosphorus: 156mg
- Carbohydrates: 47g

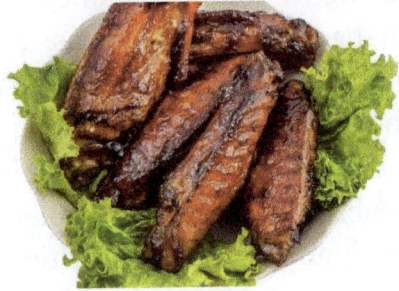

Steps

- Preheat the oven to 375°F.
- Score the dried wings on both sides with a knife.
- Rub the wings with the spice rub, making them penetrate the slits.
- Place the wings on a baking tray, cover them, and bake for 30 minutes.
- Remove the foil, flip the wings, and cook for 30 minutes more.
- Let the wings rest for 15 minutes in the switched-off oven. Baste the wings with the
- low-sodium barbecue sauce and serve.

2. Chile Chipotle Wings

Preparation time: 30 mins

Servings: 4

Ingredients

- 1/4 cup honey
- 1/4 cup slightly soft butter
- 1 lb. jumbo chicken wings, divided
- 1 tbsp. green onions, chopped
- 1 tsp. black pepper
- 1 1/2 tbsp. chopped chipotle peppers in adobo sauce
- 1 tbsp. olive oil

Nutritional facts per serving

- Calories: 384cal
- Fat: 27g
- Sodium: 100mg
- Protein: 21g
- Potassium: 267mg
- Phosphorus: 147mg
- Carbohydrates: 19g

Steps

- Preheat the oven to 400°F.
- Place the divided chicken wings on a large nonstick baking tray. Add the olive oil and toss.
- Cook the wings on the oven for around 20 minutes, turning when they become crispy on one side.
- In a wide dish, combine the other ingredients and mix thoroughly until combined.
- Remove the wings from the oven and toss them in the seasoning until properly coated.
- Serve hot.

3. Cornbread Muffins & Lime Cardamom Butter

Preparation time: 40 mins

Servings: 12

Ingredients

- 3 tbsps. lime juice
- 2 tbsps. honey
- 1 tbsp. vanilla extract
- 1 1/2 stick soft butter
- 1 egg
- 1 cup milk
- 1 cup flour
- 1 cup cornmeal
- 1 1/2 tsp. baking soda
- 1/2 tsp. lime zest
- 1/2 tsp. orange extract
- 1/4 tsp. powdered cardamom

Nutritional facts per serving

- Calories: 209cal
- Fat: 14g
- Sodium: 180mg
- Protein: 4g
- Potassium: 88mg
- Phosphorus: 68mg
- Carbohydrates: 21g

Steps

- Preheat the oven to 350°F.
- Prepare the lime cardamom butter: in a bowl whisk 1 stick of softened butter, honey, lime zest, orange extract and cardamom until they are well combined.
- Mix the cornmeal, flour, and baking soda. In a separate bowl mix the egg, milk and 1/2 softened stick of butter, beating thoroughly.
- Then, proceed to fold the dried ingredients into the liquid ingredients making sure not to over mix.
- Coat the muffin tins with nonstick spray, and then proceed to fill each cup until it is three-quarters full. Bake the muffins for around 15/18 minutes.
- Serve the hot muffins with the lime cardamom butter.

4. Protein Chocolate Smothie

Preparation time: 5 mins

Servings: 4

Ingredients

- 1 pinch of nutmeg
- 1 pinch of cinnamon
- 2 scoops of chocolate whey protein
- 2 cups ice
- 1/2 cup evaporated milk
- 1/4 cup condensed milk
- 2 tbsps. Chocolate liqueur (optional)

Nutritional Facts per Serving

- Calories: 143cal
- Fat: 5g
- Sodium: 134mg
- Protein: 11g
- Potassium: 248mg
- Phosphorus: 163mg
- Carbohydrates: 18g

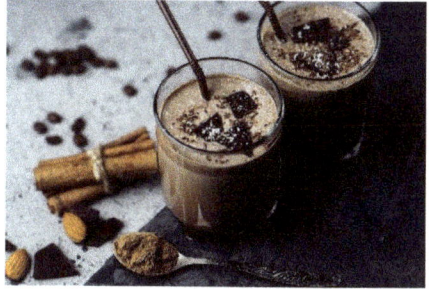

Steps

- In a food processor, mix everything together (except for the cinnamon) for around two minutes.
- Serve in glasses and sprinkle with cinnamon as a garnish.

5. Buffalo Chicken Cucumber Salad

Preparation time: 40 mins

Servings: 8

Ingredients

- 4 tbsps. crumbled blue cheese
- 4 tbsps. chopped parsley
- 1/2 cup mayonnaise
- 1/2 tsp. black pepper
- 1/2 tsp. Italian seasoning
- 1 tbsp. chopped garlic
- 1 tsp. cayenne pepper
- 1 tsp. smoked paprika
- 2 large cucumbers
- 3 tbsps. fresh chives, chopped
- 2 tbsps. hot sauce
- 2 tbsps. lemon juice
- 3 cups shredded chicken breast

Nutritional facts per serving

- Calories: 156cal
- Fat: 14g
- Sodium: 253mg
- Protein: 19g
- Potassium: 284mg
- Phosphorus: 160mg
- Carbohydrates: 5g

Steps

- Scoop out the center of the cucumbers and discard. Cut in slices.
- In a bowl, mix all the ingredients together, except the cucumbers and chicken.
- Stir in the chicken and mix until it is well coated before refrigerating for about 30 minutes.
- Place the cucumber slices on a serving plate, pour the chicken mix over and garnish with parsley.

6. Crispy Cauliflower Phyllo Cups

Preparation time: 25 mins

Servings: 24

Ingredients

- 4 slices bacon
- 3 phyllo dough sheets
- 3 eggs
- 2 tbsps. chopped jalapeños
- 2 tbsps. butter
- 1 1/2 cups cooked cauliflower florets
- 1 tbsp. mint
- 1/2 tsp. hot pepper flakes
- 1/2 tsp. ground black pepper
- 1 cup shredded cheddar cheese
- 4 tbsps. cup spring onions, finely diced
- 1 pinch black pepper

Nutritional facts per serving

- Calories: 69cal
- Fat: 6g
- Sodium: 108mg
- Protein: 4g
- Potassium: 43mg
- Phosphorus: 50mg
- Carbohydrates: 3g

Steps

- Preheat the oven to 375°F.
- Scramble the eggs in a pan with 1 tbsp of olive oil. Remove and set aside.
- Melt the butter in the same pan. Sauté the diced bacon until crispy. Add the spring onions, onions, jalapeños, cauliflower, and hot pepper flakes and sauté until the onions becomes caramelized. Season with ground black pepper and mint.
- Add the cheese of the pan, turn the heat off and let cool.

- Take each phyllo sheet and cut them into 24 square-shaped pieces (total 72 pieces) and layer them 3 by 3 them into a mini muffin tin pan.
- Fill each muffin cup with equal quantities of the mixture and bake around 15 minutes or until the edges of the phyllo become slightly crispy. Take out of the oven, let cool for a couple of minutes and serve.

7. Cereal Protein Bars

Preparation time: 20 mins

Servings: 12

Ingredients

- 2 1/2 cups toasted rolled oats
- 1 cup dried cranberries
- 4 oz. crunchy peanut butter
- 4 oz. cup honey
- 4 oz. cup flaxseeds
- 4 oz. cup cashews

Nutritional facts per serving

- Calories: 284cal
- Fat: 14g
- Sodium: 50mg
- Protein: 8g
- Potassium: 259mg
- Phosphorus: 178mg
- Carbohydrates: 40g

Steps

- Toast the oats in a hot pan about 10 minutes at they turn golden brown.
- Mix all the ingredients together in a bowl.
- Put a sheet of parchment paper on a plate; pour the mix and try to shape a loaf. Wrap and then refrigerate for a minimum of one hour or overnight.
- Cut the protein bars into the desired shape and serve.

8. Homemade Savory Biscuits

Preparation time: 30 mins

Servings: 12

Ingredients

- 4 tbsps. cup mayonnaise
- 1/2 tsp baking soda
- 6 oz. cup skimmed milk
- 1 tsp. cream of tartar
- 1 3/4 cups all-purpose flour
- 1 tbsp. fresh chopped parsley
- 1 tbsp. fresh chopped rosemary
- 1 tbsp. fresh chopped chives
- Non-stick cooking spray

Nutritional facts per serving

- Calories: 110cal
- Fat: 5g
- Sodium: 89mg
- Protein: 4g
- Potassium: 86mg
- Phosphorus: 35mg
- Carbohydrates: 16g

Steps

- Preheat the oven to 350°F. Then, apply non-stick cooking spray to a baking sheet.
- Mix the flour, cream of tartar and baking soda in a bowl. Then, mix in the mayonnaise until the paste looks like coarse cornmeal.
- Add the milk and herbs to the flour mixture and mix well.
- Spoon the mix on the baking sheet and bake for about 12 minutes or until golden brown.
- Serve the biscuits immediately or refrigerate.

9. Angel's Deviled Eggs

Preparation time: 20 mins

Servings: 4

Ingredients

- 4 large eggs (hard-boiled and peeled)
- 2 tbsps. light mayonnaise
- 1 tbsp. onion, finely chopped
- 1/2 tsp. apple cider vinegar
- 1/2 tsp. dry mustard
- 1/2 tsp. ground black pepper
- 1 pinch of smoked paprika

Nutritional facts per serving

- Calories: 99cal
- Fat: 8g
- Sodium: 125mg
- Protein: 7g
- Potassium: 74mg
- Phosphorus: 91mg
- Carbohydrates: 3g

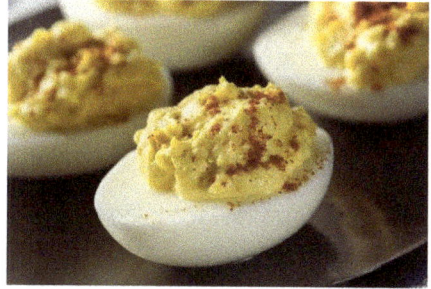

Steps

- Cut the eggs in half lengthwise. Spoon out the yolks and place the egg whites on a tray.
- Mash the yolks with a fork adding the dried mustard, onion, vinegar, mayonnaise and black pepper.
- Refill the half egg whites with the seasoned yolk mixture.
- Refrigerate and serve sprinkling with smoked paprika.

10. Beef Jerky

Preparation time: 40 mins

Servings: 30

Ingredients

- 1 1/2 tsps. Worcestershire sauce
- 1 tsp. garlic powder
- 1 tsp. hot pepper sauce
- 1/2 cup red dry wine
- 4 tbsps. dark brown sugar
- 2 tbsps. liquid smoke
- 1 tbsp. Tabasco sauce
- 3 lb. flank steak (or other lean meat)
- 1/2 cup low-sodium soy sauce

Nutritional facts per serving

- Calories: 101cal
- Fat: 8g
- Sodium: 101mg
- Protein: 13g
- Potassium: 102mg
- Phosphorus: 191mg
- Carbohydrates: 5g

Steps

- Trim or remove all the fat from the meat.
- Cut it lengthwise into 30 long strips along the grain.
- Place the strips in a mixing bowl.
- Whisk all the other ingredients together and pour them over the meat. Allow the meat to marinate for six hours or overnight in the refrigerator.
- Remove the meat from the marinade and pat dry with kitchen paper.
- If you have a dehydrator, dry out the meat for about 5 to 20 hours at 145°F.
- Otherwise, Preheat the oven to 175°F, place a baking sheet over the wire rack and distribute the meat, ensuring that the strips do not overlap.
- Bake the beef for 10 to 12 hours until it is very dry and brittle.

11. Edamame Guacamole

Preparation time: 20 mins

Servings: 6

Ingredients

- 3/4 cup frozen green soybeans or edamame (thawed)
- 3 tbsps. water
- 2 tbsps. olive oil
- 1/4 cup chopped parsley leaves
- 1 tbsp. lemon zest
- 1 tbsp. lemon juice
- 1 garlic clove
- 1/4 tsp. hot sauce

Nutritional facts per serving

- Calories: 75cal
- Fat: 2g
- Sodium: 6mg
- Protein: 4g
- Potassium: 143mg
- Phosphorus: 39mg
- Carbohydrates: 4g

Steps

- Put all the ingredients in a food processor and pulse until the mixture becomes smooth.
- Cover and refrigerate.
- Serve with tortilla chips or wedges of pita (next recipe).

12. Savory Pita Wedges

Preparation time: 15 mins

Servings: 8

Ingredients

- tsp. dried rosemary
- 1/2 cup parmesan cheese, grated
- 4 rounds pita bread
- 4 tbsps. melted unsalted butter

Nutritional facts per serving

- Calories: 105cal
- Fat: 6g
- Sodium: 162mg
- Protein: 4g
- Potassium: 31mg
- Phosphorus: 46mg
- Carbohydrates: 12g

Steps

- Brush 1 tbsp. of butter each over the pita bread.
- Cut each bread into 8 pieces and sprinkle with rosemary and parmesan.
- Toast the bread in an oven at 450°F until the cheese melts, 3 to 5 minutes.
- You may serve the pita wedges with edamame guacamole (previous recipe).

13. Rosemary Sage Crackers

Preparation time: 25 mins

Servings: 12

Ingredients

- 3 tbsps. vegetable oil
- 2 tbsps. and 1/3 cup parmesan cheese, grated
- 1/3 cup buckwheat flour
- 1/2 cup water
- 1 tsp. garlic powder
- 1 tbsp. sage, finely chopped
- 1 tbsp. rosemary, finely chopped
- 1 tbsp. olive oil
- 1 1/4 cups all-purpose flour

Nutritional facts per serving

- Calories: 110cal
- Fat: 4g
- Sodium: 39mg
- Protein: 4g
- Potassium: 35mg
- Phosphorus: 44mg
- Carbohydrates: 14g

Steps

- Preheat the oven to 350°F.
- In a medium-sized dish, mix all-purpose flour, minced rosemary and sage, buckwheat flour, and two tablespoons of parmesan cheese.
- Make a well in the center of the flour mixture.
- Pour the water and 3 tbsps. of vegetable oil into the well and mix everything together.
- Knead the dough with a rolling pin until it is less than one-eighth of an inch thick.
- Put the dough on a baking sheet and cut through the dough to make one-inch-long squares.
- Brush each square the dough with 1 tbsp. olive oil.
- Sprinkle some garlic powder and parmesan cheese on top.

- Bake until the dough is crispy or light brown, around 15 to 20 minutes.
- Divide the dough into individual crackers and serve

14. Rhubarb Cooler

Preparation time: 5 mins

Servings: 8

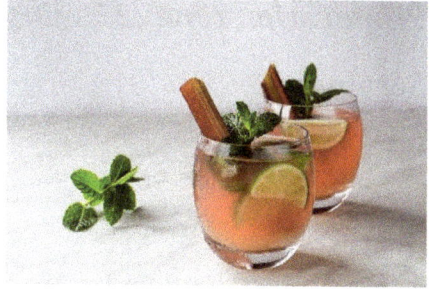

Ingredients

- 8 cups water
- 1/3 cup dark sugar
- Fresh mint leaves
- 1 lime cut in 8 wedges
- 8 chopped rhubarb stalks

Nutritional facts per serving

- Calories: 44cal
- Fat: 0g
- Sodium: 2mg
- Protein: 0g
- Potassium: 148mg
- Phosphorus: 8mg
- Carbohydrates: 12g

Steps

- Boil the stalks in the water for about 1 hour.
- Strain the liquid, add the sugar and stir thoroughly until dissolved.
- Let cool in the fridge.
- Put ice into tall glasses and pour the tea.
- Garnish with lime wedges, mint leaves and serve.

15. Rhubarb Lemonade Punch

Preparation time: 25 mins

Servings: 6

Ingredients

- 6 oz. frozen lemonade concentrate
- 5 tbsps. dark sugar
- 2 cups lemonade soda
- 3 cups of frozen rhubarb
- 3 cups water

Nutritional facts per serving

- Calories: 135cal
- Fat: 0g
- Sodium: 12mg
- Protein: 2g
- Potassium: 144mg
- Phosphorus: 17mg
- Carbohydrates: 35g

Steps

- In a pot mix all the ingredients, except the soda.
- Cover and simmer until the rhubarb becomes tender, around half an hour.
- Strain and let the liquid cool in the refrigerator
- Just before serving, put ice in tall glasses, pour the rhubarb mixture over the ice and top with chilled soda.

16. Hot Apple Punch

Preparation time: 15 mins

Servings: 8

Ingredients

- 2 quarts apple juice
- 1/2 tsp. cloves
- 2 cinnamon sticks
- 1 tsp. allspice
- 1 pinch nutmeg

Nutritional facts per serving

- Calories: 115cal
- Fat: 0g
- Sodium: 29mg
- Protein: 0g
- Potassium: 256mg
- Phosphorus: 2mg
- Carbohydrates: 29g

Steps

- Heat the apple over medium heat
- Add the remaining ingredients and bring the mixture to a simmer for around 10 minutes.
- Strain the cider into mugs and serve hot or pour into a thermos for later use.

17. Moose Jerky

Preparation time: 2 hours

Servings: 22

Ingredients

- 3 lbs. rump moose meat
- 2 tsps. liquid smoke
- 1/2 tsp. ground black pepper
- 1/2 tsp. powdered onion
- 1/2 tsp. powdered garlic
- 1/4 cup low-sodium soy sauce

Nutritional facts per serving

- Calories: 69cal
- Fat: 1g
- Sodium: 202mg
- Protein: 15g
- Potassium: 199mg
- Phosphorus: 103mg
- Carbohydrates: 1g

Steps

- Trim all the fat from the meat and cut into half-inch-thick strips.
- Whisk all the marinade ingredients in a bowl. Add the meat strips, mix well and let it marinate in the fridge for six hours.
- Proceed to preheat the oven to 180°F.
- Use parchment paper to cover a tray; spread the meat strips on the tray and cook for around two hours.
- Switch the heat off, let the meat cool in the oven and serve.

18. Baba Ghanouj

Preparation time: 30 mins

Servings: 8

Ingredients

- 8 large, unpeeled garlic cloves
- 1 large eggplant
- 2 tbsps. olive oil
- Lemon juice
- 1tbsp. chopped parsley
- 1/2 tsp. black ground pepper

Nutritional facts per serving

- Calories: 52cal
- Fat: 4g
- Sodium: 3mg
- Protein: 2g
- Potassium: 171mg
- Phosphorus: 23mg
- Carbohydrates: 6g

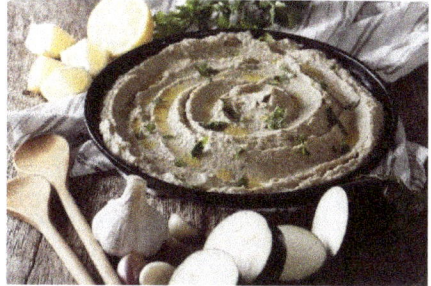

Steps

- Heat the oven to 350°F. Line a baking tray with parchment paper.
- Cut the eggplant in half and place the halves on the tray, cut side down.
- Cutoff the garlic cloves ends, place them on an aluminum foil, close the packet and put it on the baking tray.
- Roast the eggplant and garlic; after 20 minutes take the garlic packet out of the oven. Cook the eggplant until the flesh becomes very soft, around 40 more minutes.
- Turn the oven off, let the eggplant cool and remove

the skin. Open the garlic packet and remove the garlic skin.

- Place the garlic, eggplant flesh, oil, lemon juice and parsley in a food processor. Pulse until smooth and season with ground black pepper.
- Serve with pita bread.

19. Spicy Eggplant Dip

Preparation time: 1 hour

Servings: 6

Ingredients

- 1 medium eggplant
- 1 tsp. olive oil
- 1 tbsp. lemon juice
- 1/4 cup fresh coriander
- 1/4 tsp. hot pepper flakes
- 1 tbsp. chopped garlic
- 1 tbsp. chopped green onions

Nutritional facts per serving

- Calories: 24cal
- Fat: 1g
- Sodium: 3mg
- Protein: 2g
- Potassium: 199mg
- Phosphorus: 24mg
- Carbohydrates: 6g

Steps

- Preheat the oven at 350°F
- Cut the eggplant in half, drizzle with olive oil. Roast the eggplant cut face down on a baking tray lined with parchment paper. When the eggplant is very tender, around 1 hour, turn the oven off.
- Let the eggplant cool and discard the skin.
- In a food processor, mix all the ingredients together until they become smooth.
- Serve with pita bread or crackers.

20. Spicy Crab Dip

Preparation time: 20 mins

Servings: 6

Ingredients

- 6 oz. crab meat
- 1 cup soft cream cheese
- 1 tbsp. spring onion, chopped
- 1 tsp. lemon juice
- 1 pinch ground black pepper
- 2 tbsps. cream
- 2 tsps. low-sodium soy sauce
- 1/2 tsp. hot pepper flakes

Nutritional facts per serving

- Calories: 99cal
- Fat: 10g
- Sodium: 133mg
- Protein: 6g
- Potassium: 92mg
- Phosphorus: 62mg
- Carbohydrates: 3g

Steps

- Preheat the oven to 375°F.
- In a bowl, mix with a spoon the cream cheese, spring onion, soy sauce, lemon juice, hot pepper, and black pepper. Add the cream, crab meat and mix thoroughly.
- Place the mixture in a baking dish and bake uncovered for around for 15 minutes, until the surface of the mix is sizzling. Serve with crackers or pita bread.

21. Crab Pies

Preparation time: 20 mins

Servings: 8

Ingredients

- 1 tbsps. olive oil
- 2 tbsps. parsley, chopped
- 4 tbsps. green onions, chopped
- 1 pinch ground black pepper
- 4 oz. crab meat
- 1/4 cup green peppers, diced
- 1/4 cup panko breadcrumbs
- 1 tsp. lemon juice
- 1 egg, beaten
- 1 garlic clove, chopped

Nutritional facts per serving

- Calories: 76cal
- Fat: 6g
- Sodium: 89mg
- Protein: 6g
- Potassium: 117mg
- Phosphorus: 61mg
- Carbohydrates: 5g

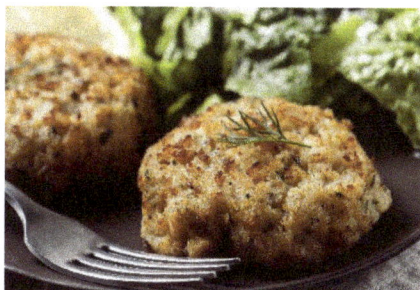

Steps

- Mix all the ingredients except the olive oil in a mixing bowl.
- Divide the mixture into eight equal parts.
- Shape the crab cakes by hand and place them on a tray.
- Heat the olive oil in a wide pan and fry the crab cakes on each side for about two minutes or until they are golden brown.
- Serve immediately.

22. Cream Cheese Spread

Preparation time: 10 mins

Servings: 5

Ingredients

- 20 slices toasted bread
- 2 tbsps. water
- 2 tbsps. spring onions, minced
- 1 cup soft cream cheese
- 1 garlic clove
- 1/2 tsp. freshly ground black pepper
- 1/4 cup mixed chopped fresh parsley, dill, and thyme

Nutritional facts per serving

- Calories: 80cal
- Fat: 3g
- Sodium: 173mg
- Protein: 3g
- Potassium: 63mg
- Phosphorus: 48mg
- Carbohydrates: 11g

Steps

- In a blender, mix the cheese, water, herbs, spring onions, pepper.
- Rub the garlic clove on the toasted bread slices.
- Spread the mixture on the bread and serve.

23. Spicy Nacho Chips

Preparation time: 15 mins

Servings: 24

Ingredients

- 12 cups unsalted nacho chips
- 6 tbsps. margarine
- 2 tbsps. low-sodium soy sauce
- 1tsp. powdered garlic
- 1 tsp. dried oregano
- 1/2 tsp. powder onion
- 1 tsp. smoked paprika
- 1 pinch hot pepper

Nutritional facts per serving

- Calories: 91cal
- Fat: 4g
- Sodium: 191mg
- Protein: 2g
- Potassium: 45mg
- Phosphorus: 26mg
- Carbohydrates: 15g

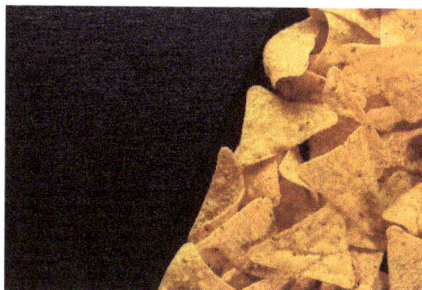

Steps

- Heat the oven to 250 °F.
- In a skillet, melt the margarine. Add all the seasoning and mix well.
- In a big bowl, toss the nacho chips with the seasoner margarine. Mix well co coat all the chips in the seasoning.
- Distribute the chips on a wide baking tray and bake for about 15 minutes.

24. Bannock Bread

Preparation time: 50 mins

Servings: 24

Ingredients

- 3 tsps. baking soda
- 5 cups water
- 1 cup and 2 tbsps. Unsalted margarine
- 4 tsps. cream of tartar
- 10 cups white flour

Nutritional facts per serving

- Calories: 270cal
- Fat: 10g
- Sodium: 85mg
- Protein: 6g
- Potassium: 141mg
- Phosphorus: 58mg
- Carbohydrates: 41g

Steps

- Preheat the oven to 350°F.
- Stir all the dry ingredients together and add the water and 1 cup of melted margarine, little by little, kneading until you get a ball of dough.
- Cover with cling film and let rest for 30 minutes.
- Knead for 10 more minutes and divide the dough in 2 parts.
- Shape the dough balls into flat breads and put them into 2 10" round baking tins.
- With a wet knife, score the breads to cut into wedges.
- Bake the breads for 50 minutes or until they turn golden brown.
- Take the breads out of the oven and brush a little melted margarine on top.
- Let the breads cool and serve.

25. Homemade Pickles

Preparation time: 20 mins

Servings: 30

Ingredients

- 2 cups dill, chopped
- 1 tsp. black pepper
- 1 tsp. turmeric
- 2 cups white sugar
- 2 1/2cups rice vinegar
- 2 tsps. nigella seeds
- 5 big cucumbers
- 2 1/2 cups apple cider vinegar
- 1/2 tsp. dry mustard

Nutritional facts per serving

- Calories: 30cal
- Fat: 0g
- Sodium: 1mg
- Protein: 0g
- Potassium: 16mg
- Phosphorus: 2mg
- Carbohydrates: 9g

Steps

- Slice and divide the cucumbers into quart-sized jars, adding the nigella seeds and chopped dill between layers.
- Thoroughly whisk the sugar, turmeric, mustard, pepper and vinegars in a pitcher until the sugar is completely dissolved.
- Pour the mix in the jars, close and refrigerate for at least 1 month before serving.

26. Ginger Cranberry Cooler

Preparation time: 10 mins

Servings: 60

Ingredients

- 6 cups cranberry juice
- 6 tbsps. fresh ginger
- 1/2 cup fresh lime juice
- 1/2 cup granulated sugar

Nutritional facts per serving

- Calories: 125cal
- Fat: 0g
- Sodium: 1mg
- Protein: 1g
- Potassium: 51mg
- Phosphorus: 1mg
- Carbohydrates: 32g

Steps

- Thinly slice the fresh ginger.
- Bring to a simmer the cranberry juice and ginger in a pot, for about 20 minutes.
- Let cool, then add the lime juice and sugar, and whisk until the sugar dissolve
- Strain the drink and serve over ice in tall glasses.

Desserts

1. Orange & Cinnamon Biscuits

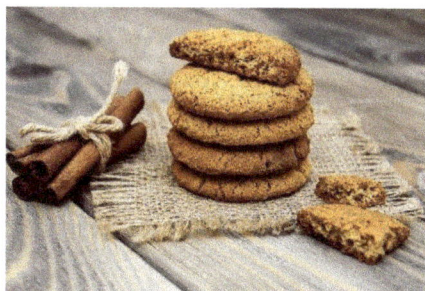

Nutritional facts per serving

- Calories: 150cal
- Fat: 7g
- Sodium: 77mg
- Protein: 3g
- Potassium: 54mg
- Phosphorus: 29mg
- Carbohydrates: 23g

Preparation time: 50 mins

Servings: 18

Ingredients

- 2 tsps. grated orange peel
- 2 large eggs
- 2 cups all-purpose flour
- 1 tsp. vanilla extract
- 1 tsp. ground cinnamon
- 1 tsp. cream of tartar
- 1 cup sugar
- 1/2 tsp. baking soda
- 1/2 cup unsalted butter, melted

Steps

- Preheat the oven to 325°F.
- Apply non-stick cooking spray to two baking sheets.
- In a large cup, mix the sugar and unsalted butter together.
- Add the eggs (one at a time), beating the mixture after each one.
- Whisk together the orange peel and the vanilla.
- In a medium-sized dish, combine the flour, cream of tartar, baking soda and cinnamon.

- Add the dry ingredients to the butter mixture and combine until blended.
- Cut the dough in two. Put each half on a sheet and shape each half into a log. Bake the dough for 35 minutes and then remove them from the oven.
- Let the bread cool for 10 minutes.
- Move the logs to the surface and cut them diagonally into half-inch-thick slices using a serrated blade.
- Proceed to bake the biscuits for 12 minutes until the bottoms become golden.
- Before serving, move them to a wire rack and allow them to cool.

2. Berry Bread Pudding

Preparation time: 50 mins

Servings: 18

Ingredients

- Whipped cream, to serve
- 8 cups cubed bread
- 6 eggs, beaten
- 2 tsps. vanilla
- 2 cups heavy cream
- 12 oz. frozen berries, thawed
- 1 tbsp. orange zest
- 1/2 tsp. cinnamon
- 1/2 cup sugar

Nutritional facts per serving

- Calories: 393cal
- Fat: 24g
- Sodium: 232mg
- Protein: 10g
- Potassium: 173mg
- Phosphorus: 134mg
- Carbohydrates 37g

Steps

- Preheat the oven to 375°F.
- Whisk together the eggs, sugar, cream, vanilla, orange zest, and cinnamon.
- Gently mix the cubes of bread and the fruit with your hands.
- Pour the cubes into a buttered or oiled up pan and bake them for 35 minutes.
- Take out the foil and cook the bread for an extra 15 minutes.
- Turn the oven off and let the bread sit for about 10 minutes.
- Cut and serve.

3. Chewy Lemon Coconut Cookies

Preparation time: 30 mins

Servings: 24

Ingredients

- 1/2 cup unsalted butter
- 1/2 cup sugar
- 1/2 tsp. baking soda
- 1 1/4 cups flour
- 1 cup toasted coconut
- 1 egg
- 1 tbsp. fresh grated ginger
- 1 tbsp. lemon zest
- 2 tbsps. lemon juice

Nutritional facts per serving

- Calories: 97cal
- Fat: 7g
- Sodium: 40mg
- Protein: 2g
- Potassium: 27mg
- Phosphorus: 17mg
- Carbohydrates: 11g

Steps

- Spread the unsweetened coconut on the baking sheet tray and bake for up to 10 minutes until the edges become light brown.
- Take it out of the oven and set it aside in a bowl.
- Mix the butter and sugar until it becomes light and fluffy with an electric mixer. Add the egg, lemon juice, lemon zest, and chopped ginger and blend until smooth.
- Sift the flour and baking soda together. Stir them in the butter mixture, whisking constantly.
- Cover the bowl and rest for a minimum of 30 minutes.
- Preheat the oven to 350°F.
- Scoop out a few tablespoons, roll them into balls, and cover them with toasted coconut flakes. Use a lightly oiled baking sheet and place the balls at a minimum of two inches apart.
- Bake them for 10 to 12 minutes or until the sides become slightly brown. Remove and allow them to cool on the counter.

4. Cranberry Dried Fruit Bars

Preparation time: 40 mins

Servings: 24

Ingredients

Crust

- 1 1/3 cups sugar
- 3/4 cup unsalted butter (1.5 sticks)
- 1 1/2 cups all-purpose flour
- Topping
- 1 cup dried cranberries
- 1 tsp. baking powder
- 1 tsp. vanilla extract
- 4 large eggs
- Powdered sugar (optional)

Nutritional facts per serving

- Calories: 191cal
- Fat: 7g
- Sodium: 34mg
- Protein: 3g
- Potassium: 28mg
- Phosphorus: 34mg
- Carbohydrates: 31g

Steps

- Preheat the oven to 350°F.
- Stir together the flour and sugar in a medium-sized bowl. Add melted unsalted butter until the mixture holds together. Pat it into a loaf and place into a 9" x 13" unoiled baking tray. Bake until it is gently browned for about 10 minutes.
- For the topping, mix the eggs, vanilla, sugar, flour, baking powder and cranberries in a medium-sized dish. Slather the topping onto the loaf. Continue baking for 20 to 25 minutes.
- While warm, cut the baked loaf into 24 bars and dust with powdered sugar.

5. Mint Chocolate Brownies

Preparation time: 30 mins

Servings: 12

Ingredients

- 1 box brownie mix
- 12 Andes mint chocolates

Nutritional facts per serving

- Calories: 308cal
- Fat: 18g
- Sodium: 146mg
- Protein: 4g
- Potassium: 120mg
- Phosphorus: 61mg
- Carbohydrates: 36g

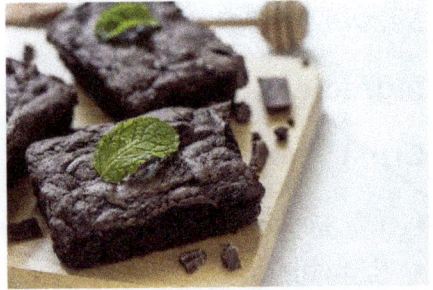

Steps

- Preheat the oven at 350°F
- Prepare lightly oiled 12-cup muffin tin and add flour to both the bottom and the sides.
- Add the brownie mix to the cups and bake for about 25 minutes.
- Place a piece of mint candy in the middle of each cup and bake for an extra 5 minutes.
- Remove the brownies from the oven. Then, turn the oven off and allow the brownies to rest for 5 to 10 minutes.
- Remove them from the tin and serve.

6. Festive Cheese Sugar Cookies

Preparation time: 30 mins

Servings: 12

Ingredients

- 1/4 tsp. almond extract
- 1/2 tsp. vanilla extract
- 1 cup unsalted butter, softened
- 1 cup sugar
- 1 large egg, separated
- 2 1/4 cups all-purpose flour
- 3 oz. cream cheese, softened
- Colored sugar for garnishing

Nutritional facts per serving

- Calories: 80cal
- Fat: 6g
- Sodium: 34mg
- Protein: 2g
- Potassium: 12mg
- Phosphorus: 11mg
- Carbohydrates: 10g

Steps

- Mix the sugar, butter, almond extract, cream cheese, vanilla extract, and egg yolk in a large bowl. Then, add flour and whisk it in.
- Refrigerate the cookie dough for two hours.
- Proceed to preheat the oven to 350°F.
- Roll the dough on a floured surface and cut it into the desired shapes using cookie cutters.
- Place them one inch apart on unoiled cookie sheets. Keep the cookies plain or, if desired, brush them with the beaten egg white and sprinkle with colored sugar.
- Bake the cream cheese cookies for about seven to nine minutes or until they become light golden brown. Let them cool before serving.

7. Yellow Cake

Preparation time: 30 mins

Servings: 8

Ingredients

- 1 egg
- 1 1/2 cups of Master Mix
- 1/2 cup water
- 1/2 tsp. vanilla
- 2/3 cup sugar

Nutritional facts per serving

- Calories: 340cal
- Fat: 12g
- Sodium: 406mg
- Protein: 5g
- Potassium: 53mg
- Phosphorus: 225mg
- Carbohydrates: 72g

Steps

- Preheat the oven to 375°F.
- Use the Master Mix recipe and add sugar to the blend.
- In a separate dish, combine the water, egg, and vanilla.
- Pour half the liquid into the Master Mix contents and stir for two minutes.
- Then, add the remainder of the liquid and whisk everything together for two more minutes.
- Bake the cake for 25 minutes in a pan lined with parchment paper.

8. Sweet Berries & Mascarpone

Preparation time: 20 mins

Servings: 6

Ingredients

- 1 cup of diced strawberries
- 1 tbsp. lemon or orange zest
- 1/2 cup and 2 tsps. sugar
- 1/4 cup marsala wine or balsamic vinegar
- 2 cups mascarpone cheese

Nutritional facts per serving

- Calories: 754cal
- Fat: 9g
- Sodium: 82mg
- Protein: 12g
- Potassium: 119mg
- Phosphorus: 19mg
- Carbohydrates: 25g

Steps

- Mix the cheese, citrus zest, and 1/2 cup sugar together until they become smooth.
- Mix the berries and the balsamic vinegar with the sugar and leave it to rest for a minimum of 10 minutes.
- Divide the berries into the dessert cups and cover each with the cheese.

9. Angel Food Cake

Preparation time: 25 mins

Servings: 12

- Potassium: 124mg
- Phosphorus: 132mg
- Carbohydrates: 36g

Ingredients

- tbsp. granulated sugar
- 1 package Angel Food cake mix
- 1/2 tsp. lemon zest
- 1/2 tsp. vanilla extract
- 1/2 pint heavy whipping cream
- 7,5 oz. chopped canned peaches (reserve the juice)
- 7,5 oz chopped canned pineapple crushed (reserve the juice)

Nutritional facts per serving

- Calories: 217cal
- Fat: 4g
- Sodium: 262mg
- Protein: 5g

Steps

- Use the reserved juices and mix with the cake mix, in accordance with the package's directions.
- If the juice is not enough, add water.
- Fold the canned fruit into the mix and then bake according to the package's instructions.
- Use an electric mixer to combine the remaining ingredients and whisk everything until the desired consistency is achieved.
- Serve the cake with whipped cream.

10. Easy Cheesecake

Preparation time: 3 hours

Servings: 8

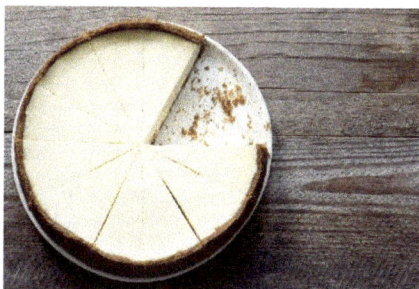

Ingredients

- 4 eggs
- 2 packs crushed crackers
- 16 oz. cream cheese, softened
- 1/2 cup sugar
- 1 tbsp. vanilla extract
- 1 stick unsalted butter, softened

Nutritional facts per serving

- Calories: 126cal
- Fat: 6g
- Sodium: 228mg
- Protein: 9g
- Potassium: 175mg
- Phosphorus: 80mg
- Carbohydrates: 13g

Steps

- Preheat the oven to 325°F.
- Mix the butter and the crushed crackers until they are completely combined. Spread the mixture evenly on the bottom of a pan.
- Whisk the cream cheese, eggs, sugar, and vanilla until they are completely mixed. Pour the mixture onto the crust. Proceed to bake the cake for about 45 to 60 minutes or until the center no longer jiggles.
- Let the mixture cool for three hours.
- Try topping with your favorite sauce.

11. Strawberries Brulèe

Preparation time: 10 mins

Servings: 8

Ingredients

- 6 oz. of cream cheese
- 1/4 cup and 2 tbsps. brown sugar, divided and packed
- 1 quart fresh strawberries
- 1 cup sour cream

Nutritional facts per serving

- Calories: 188cal
- Fat: 8g
- Sodium: 69mg
- Protein: 4g
- Potassium: 208mg
- Phosphorus: 60mg
- Carbohydrates: 10g

Steps

- Blend the cream cheese with an electric mixer until it softens. Then, add two tablespoons of brown sugar and the sour cream. Beat until they become smooth.
- Cut the strawberries in half and arrange them uniformly in a shallow, circular, eight-inch-long broilerproof dish.
- Cover the berries with the cream mixture.
- Sprinkle the leftover quarter cup of brown sugar over the cream mixture.
- Broil for one to two minutes or until the sugar becomes golden brown.
- Serve immediately.

12. Squash Cookies

Preparation time: 20 mins

Servings: 30

Ingredients

- 1 1/2 cups cooked winter squash, mashed
- 1 1/2 cups pecans or walnuts, chopped
- 1 cup raisins
- 1 tsp. baking soda
- 1 tsp. cinnamon
- 1/2 cup softened butter
- 1/2 tsp. ground cardamom
- 1/4 tsp. allspice
- 1/4 tsp. ground ginger
- 2 1/2 cups flour
- 2 1/2 tsps. baking powder
- 2 eggs
- 1 1/2 cups brown sugar

Nutritional facts per serving

- Calories: 85cal
- Fat: 4g
- Sodium: 126mg
- Protein: 3g
- Potassium: 161mg
- Phosphorus: 55mg
- Carbohydrates: 8g

Steps

- Preheat the oven to 375°F.
- Mix the butter and sugar until they become fluffy.
- Beat the eggs together.
- Then, mix together the dry ingredients and stir in the eggs, butter and sugar; add the mashed squash to the mixture.
- Whisk in the nuts and raisins.
- Spoon the mixture onto a baking sheet and bake for 10 to 12 minutes.

13. Vanilla Cream Sauce

Preparation time: 30 mins

Servings: 6

Ingredients

- 1 1/2 cups milk
- 1 vanilla bean, halved lengthwise
- 2 tbsps. cornstarch
- 3 egg yolks
- 3 tbsps. of granulated sugar
- 2 tbsps. brandy (optional)

Nutritional facts per serving

- Calories: 68.8cal
- Fat: 0.6g
- Sodium: 51.8mg
- Protein: 2.1g
- Potassium: 112mg
- Phosphorus: 87mg
- Carbohydrates: 33.8g

Steps

- Use two beans if you are recycling vanilla beans from a different recipe.
- Use a sharp knife to scrape the pods off the vanilla bean and put them in a small saucepan with the milk.
- Allow the milk to simmer at medium-high heat but do not let it boil. Continue to stir occasionally.
- Remove the milk from the heat and let it cool.
- Whisk in the milk the egg yolks, and cornstarch.
- Boil the milk over high heat, constantly whisking.
- Check the mixture with the back of a spoon and see if it becomes coated with a thin layer. If yes, this indicates that it's thickening. Once it thickens, it should be ready.
- Pour the sauce quickly in a ceramic or metal bowl and let it cool and reach room temperature, stirring occasionally.
- You can add the liquor to it when the cream cools (if desired).

14. Rhubarb Pie

Preparation time: 1 hour

Servings: 8

Ingredients

- 4 cups unpeeled rhubarb stalks, diced
- 2 eggs
- 1/4 cup flour
- 1 tsp. grated orange rind
- 1 tbsp. butter
- 1 recipe pie crust (double crust)
- 2 cups sugar

Nutritional facts per serving

- Calories: 386cal
- Fat: 10g
- Sodium: 121mg
- Protein: 3g
- Potassium: 90mg
- Phosphorous: 21mg
- Carbohydrates: 21g

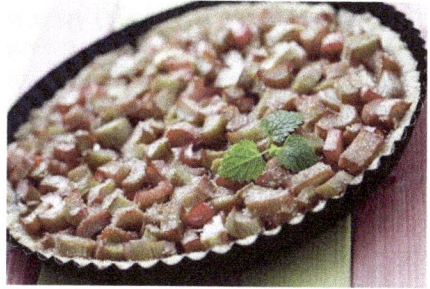

Steps

- Preheat the oven to 450°F.
- Whisk eggs with butter, flour and sugar until
- it becomes very creamy and gently add the diced rhubarb.
- Let the mixture rest for 15 minutes, then pour in a pie shell.
- Sprinkle with orange rind and put the pie into the preheated oven.
- Bake for about 10 minutes, and then reduce the heat to 350°F, letting the pie bake for another 45 minutes.
- Take the pie out of the oven, let cool and serve.

15. Raspberry Bavarian Pie

Preparation time: 30 mins

Servings: 12

Ingredients

- 2 egg whites
- 2 1/2 tbsps. sugar
- 10 oz. fresh raspberries, mashed
- 1/4 tsp. vanilla
- 1/4 tsp. almond extract
- 1/3 cup butter
- 1/3 cup chopped almonds
- 1 tbsp. lemon juice
- 1 egg yolk
- 1 cup sugar
- 1 cup whipping cream
- 1 cup flour

Nutritional facts per serving

- Calories: 268cal
- Fat: 4g
- Sodium: 60mg
- Protein: 4g
- Potassium: 77mg
- Phosphorus: 39mg
- Carbohydrates: 33g

Steps

- Preheat the oven to 400°F.
- Oil a 10-inch pie pan.
- Whisk the butter with 2 1/2 tablespoons of sugar until the mixture becomes fluffy.
- Add the egg yolk and thoroughly mix everything together, before adding the flour and almonds.
- In a prepared pie pan, press and bake the crust for 12 minutes.
- Place the rest of the ingredients in a large bowl for the filling, with the exception of whipping cream.
- Beat the mixture until it thickens and increases in volume.
- Whip and fold the cream into the raspberry mixture.
- Then, add it to the pastry and refrigerate it for 8 or more hours.

16. Pumpkin Mousse Pie

Preparation time: 4 hours

Servings: 8

Ingredients

- 3/4 cup milk
- 3 1/2 cups non-dairy cool whipped topping
- 1/2 cup canned pumpkin
- 1/2 tsp. ginger
- 1/2 tsp. cinnamon
- 1/2 tsp. ground cardamom
- 1 small package vanilla pudding
- 1 baked, cooled pie shell

Nutritional facts per serving

- Calories: 239cal
- Fat: 9g
- Sodium: 295mg
- Protein: 3g
- Potassium: 111mg
- Phosphorus: 129mg
- Carbohydrates: 31g

Steps

- Add the milk to the pudding mix and beat it for about two minutes or until it thickens.
- Mix in the pumpkin and the spices.
- Proceed to fold the cool whip into two cups of the whipped topping and spread the mixture into the pie shell.
- Refrigerate it for at least four hours. Serve with the remaining cool whip.

17. Popcorn Balls

Preparation time: 20 mins

Servings: 18

Ingredients

- 1 tsp. butter
- 1 tsp. vinegar
- 2 cups sugar
- 1 tsp. vanilla
- 1 1/2 cups water
- 1/2 cup light corn syrup
- 4 quarts of popped popcorn
- 1 tsp. butter for making the balls

Nutritional facts per serving

- Calories: 147cal
- Fat: 2g
- Sodium: 8mg
- Protein: 2g
- Potassium: 28mg
- Phosphorus: 30mg
- Carbohydrates: 37g

Steps

- Add butter to the sides of a medium-sized saucepan.
- Add water, syrup, sugar, and vinegar to the pan.
- Leave it to boil, stirring over medium-high heat, stirring occasionally.
- Remove from the heat and whisk in the vanilla.
- Place the popcorn in a large bowl and pour the syrup over it.
- Let the mixture cool until your hands are ready to handle it.
- Grease your hands and form the popcorn balls.

18 Pear Cardamom Cake

Preparation time: 40 mins

Servings: 8

Ingredients

- 1 1/2 cups all-purpose flour
- 1 1/2 tsps. low-sodium baking powder
- 1 egg
- 1 tsp. vanilla
- 1/2 cup sugar
- 1/4 cup unsalted butter
- 2 tsps. ground cardamom
- 2/3 cup unsalted butter
- 3/4 cup cream
- 3/4 cup sugar
- 4 pears

Nutritional facts per serving

- Calories: 443cal
- Fat: 4g
- Sodium: 25mg
- Protein: 6g
- Potassium: 251mg
- Phosphorus: 138mg
- Carbohydrates: 59g

Steps

- Heat the oven to 350°F.
- Peel the pears, remove the core, and cut them into quarters. In a big, non-stick pan, melt a quarter cup of butter. Stir in the 1/2 cup of sugar.
- Add the pears to the mixture.
- Cover and cook for around 15 minutes on medium-high heat, checking it periodically to prevent burning
- Meanwhile, beat two-thirds of a cup of butter and three-fourths of a cup of sugar with the electric mixer or a food processor until the mixture becomes light and fluffy.
- Stir in the vanilla and egg and cream. Mix the flour with the cardamom and baking powder. Then, fold the dry ingredients into the

egg mixture with the spatula.

- Place the pears and their sauce into a 8x9"-long glass cake pan, leaving the fruit face down. Pour the batter uniformly over the pears.
- Bake in the oven for about 20 to 25 minutes until it becomes golden brown.
- Allow the cake to cool for five minutes before cutting.
- Serve immediately or when desired.

19 Pavlova Meringue Cake

Preparation time: 3 hours

Servings: 8

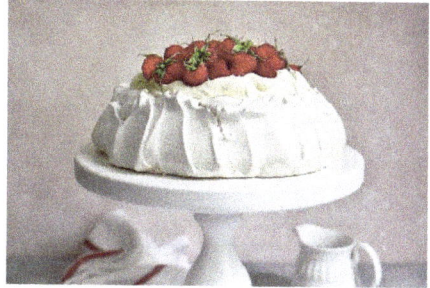

Ingredients

- 1 cup whipping cream
- 1 tbsp. cornstarch
- 1 tsp. vanilla extract
- 1 tsp. white vinegar
- 1/4 tsps. vanilla extract
- 2 cups fresh strawberries
- 2 tbsps. granulated sugar
- 3/4 cup granulated sugar
- 4 egg whites

Nutritional facts per serving

- Calories: 212cal
- Fat: 11g
- Sodium: 40mg
- Protein: 4g
- Potassium: 118mg
- Phosphorus: 30mg
- Carbohydrates: 27g

Steps

- Preheat the oven to 350°F.
- Use parchment paper to cover a cake tin.
- Beat the egg whites with an electric mixer until rigid peaks form.
- Add sugar slowly and beat for four to five minutes or until the mixture becomes stiff.
- Add 1 tsp. of vanilla extract, vinegar, and cornstarch to the egg whites and whip them until they are well mixed together.
- Spread the white egg mixture in the tin to create an 8"-wide circle, like a shallow cup, leaving the

outer edges slightly elevated.

- Place the cake batter in the oven and reduce the heat to 200°F. Leave it in the oven for one hour.
- Turn the oven off and leave the cake in it to cool for one hour with the door open.
- Whisk together two tablespoons of sugar,
- whipping cream, and 1/4 tsp. vanilla until stiff peaks are formed.
- Cover the cool meringue with the whipped cream and top with the fruit.

20. Lemon Curd

Preparation time: 20 mins

Servings: 2

Ingredients

- Zest of 4 lemons
- 4 whole eggs, well beaten
- 2/3 cup lemon juice
- 2 cups granulated sugar
- 1 cup unsalted butter

Nutritional facts per serving

- Calories: 100cal
- Fat: 3g
- Sodium: 10mg
- Protein: 2g
- Potassium: 16mg
- Phosphorus: 14mg
- Carbohydrates: 13g

Steps

- Heat the lemon juice, sugar, and zests in a saucepan until the sugar has dissolved.
- Remove the mixture from the pan and add butter. Wait for it to melt.
- When the mixture reaches room temperature, gently fold in the eggs.
- Return the mixture to the heat over a double boiler. When the mixture thickens, remove it from the heat and pour through a fine strainer.
- Refrigerate and serve.

21. Lemon Chess Pie

Preparation time: 1 hour

Servings: 8

Ingredients

- 6 tbsps. unsalted butter
- 4 large eggs
- 3 tbsps. cornstarch
- 2 tbsps. lemon zest
- 1/3 cup fresh lemon juice
- 1 cup whipped cream
- 1 sheet pie crust
- 1 1/2 cups sugar
- Fresh mint sprigs

Nutritional facts per serving

- Calories: 443cal
- Fat: 10g
- Sodium: 161mg
- Protein: 6g
- Potassium: 74mg
- Phosphorus: 70mg
- Carbohydrates: 60g

Steps

- Preheat the oven to 350°F.
- Bake a pie crust for around eight minutes or according to the box's instruction, until it becomes golden brown. Allow it to cool.
- In a large cup, beat the sugar and butter until it is light and fluffy. Then, add the lemon zest, lemon juice and cornstarch.
- Add the eggs (one at a time) and continue whisking with every addition.
- Spoon the mixture into the shell of the crust.
- Bake until the filling becomes set and the top turns golden brown (40 to 45 minutes).
- Cool and serve with whipped cream and a little sprig of mint.

22. Almond Plum Pie

Preparation time: 50 mins

Servings: 8

Ingredients

- 1/4 tsps. almond extract
- 1/2 cup sugar
- Lemon zest
- 1/2 package (4 oz.) almond paste or marzipan
- 1/2 tsp. cinnamon
- 1 pre-made pie crust
- 4 cups plums
- 6 tbsps. Cornstarch

Nutritional facts per serving

- Calories: 271cal
- Fat: 11g
- Sodium: 93mg
- Protein: 4g
- Potassium: 201mg
- Phosphorus: 67mg
- Carbohydrates: 45g

Steps

- Cut the plums in half and remove the pits.
- Combine the almond extract, sugar, lemon zest, cinnamon, cornstarch and plums in a bowl. Add the diced marzipan and mix well.
- Place the pie crust in a 9"-long dish. Pour in the filling and bake for 35 to 45 minutes at 425°F.

23. Easy Ice Cream

Preparation time: 15 mins

Servings: 4

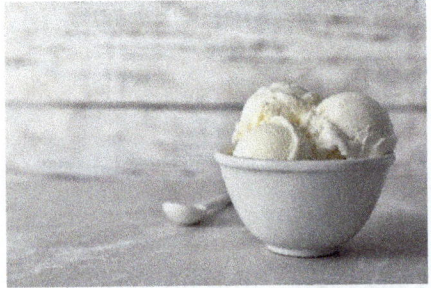

Ingredients

- 1 1/2 cups frozen fruit of your choice
- 1/2 cup sugar
- 1 cup whipping cream

Nutritional facts per serving

- Calories: 279cal
- Fat: 16g
- Sodium: 24mg
- Protein: 3g
- Potassium: 82mg
- Phosphorus: 38mg
- Carbohydrates: 22g

Steps

- Make sure the fruit is frozen (do not thaw it).
- Add all the ingredients to the food processor and pulse until the mixture becomes fluffy and very thick.
- Serve immediately.

24. Ginger Cookies

Preparation time: 20 mins

Servings: 36

Ingredients

- 3/4 cup unsalted butter
- 2 tsps. baking soda
- 2 tsps. fresh ginger (finely grated)
- 2 cups flour
- 1/4 cup dark molasses
- 1/3 cup cinnamon sugar
- 1/2 cup candied ginger (finely chopped)
- 1 tsp. cinnamon
- 1 tbsp. ground ginger
- 1 egg
- 1 cup granulated sugar

Nutritional facts per serving

- Calories: 93cal
- Fat: 4g
- Sodium: 118mg
- Protein: 2g
- Potassium: 58mg
- Phosphorus: 12mg
- Carbohydrates: 15g

Steps

- Preheat the oven to 350°F.
- In a mixing cup, combine the flour, baking soda, ginger, and cinnamon.
- Add the butter and beat until smooth. Pour in 1 cup of granulated sugar slowly, then add the molasses and egg.
- Mix thoroughly, then, add the candied ginger.
- Pinch off a small amount of the mix and roll into small balls.
- Wrap each ball in cinnamon sugar and put it on an unoiled baking sheet, two inches apart from each other.
- Bake in a preheated oven for about 10 minutes until the tops become rounded and lightly cracked.
- Allow the cookies to cool on a wire rack.
- Serve immediately or store in an air-tight jar for later.

25. Dessert Pizza

Preparation time: 20 mins

Servings: 8

Ingredients

- 1 12"-long precooked pizza crust
- 1 cup of low-fat ricotta cheese
- 1/4 cup chocolate chips
- 1/2 cup apricot jam
- 2 cups fresh sliced strawberry
- 5 tbsps. divided powdered sugar

Nutritional facts per serving

- Calories: 289cal
- Fat: 11g
- Sodium: 167mg
- Protein: 9g
- Potassium: 99mg
- Phosphorus: 48mg
- Carbohydrates: 50g

Steps

- Preheat the oven to 425°F.
- Strain the ricotta with a cheesecloth
- Heat the jam for 30 seconds in the microwave.
- Mix the ricotta with the jam, strawberries, and three teaspoons of powdered sugar.
- Pour the mix onto the pizza crust.
- Sprinkle with the chocolate chips and leftover powdered sugar.
- Bake for about 10 to 12 minutes.

26. Carrot Muffins

Preparation time: 30 mins

Servings: 12

Ingredients

- 2 large eggs
- 2 cups shredded carrots (about 6 medium-sized carrots)
- 1/2 cup all-purpose flour
- 1/2 cup whole wheat flour
- 1/2 cup oats
- 1/2 cup brown sugar
- 1/2 cup vegetable oil
- 1/2 cup unsweetened applesauce
- 3/4 tsps. baking powder
- 3/4 tsps. baking soda
- 3/4 tsps. Cinnamon

Nutritional facts per serving

- Calories: 207cal
- Fat: 13g
- Sodium: 136mg
- Protein: 5g
- Potassium: 143mg
- Phosphorus: 99mg
- Carbohydrates: 24g

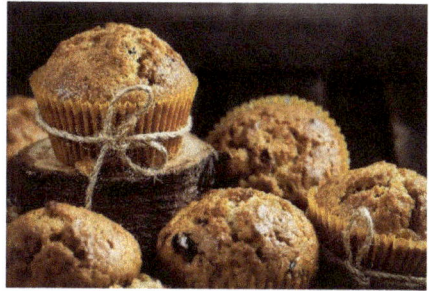

Steps

- Preheat the oven to 350°F.
- Coat the muffin tins lightly with non-stick spray.
- In a big dish, mix the dry ingredients together.
- Mix the wet ingredients in a medium-sized bowl with a whisk and then combine with the dry ingredients.
- Combine with the shredded carrots and cover the muffins with the batter.
- Bake the muffins for about 20 minutes.

CPSIA information can be obtained
at www.ICGtesting.com
Printed in the USA
LVHW081642280621
691357LV00003B/67